2

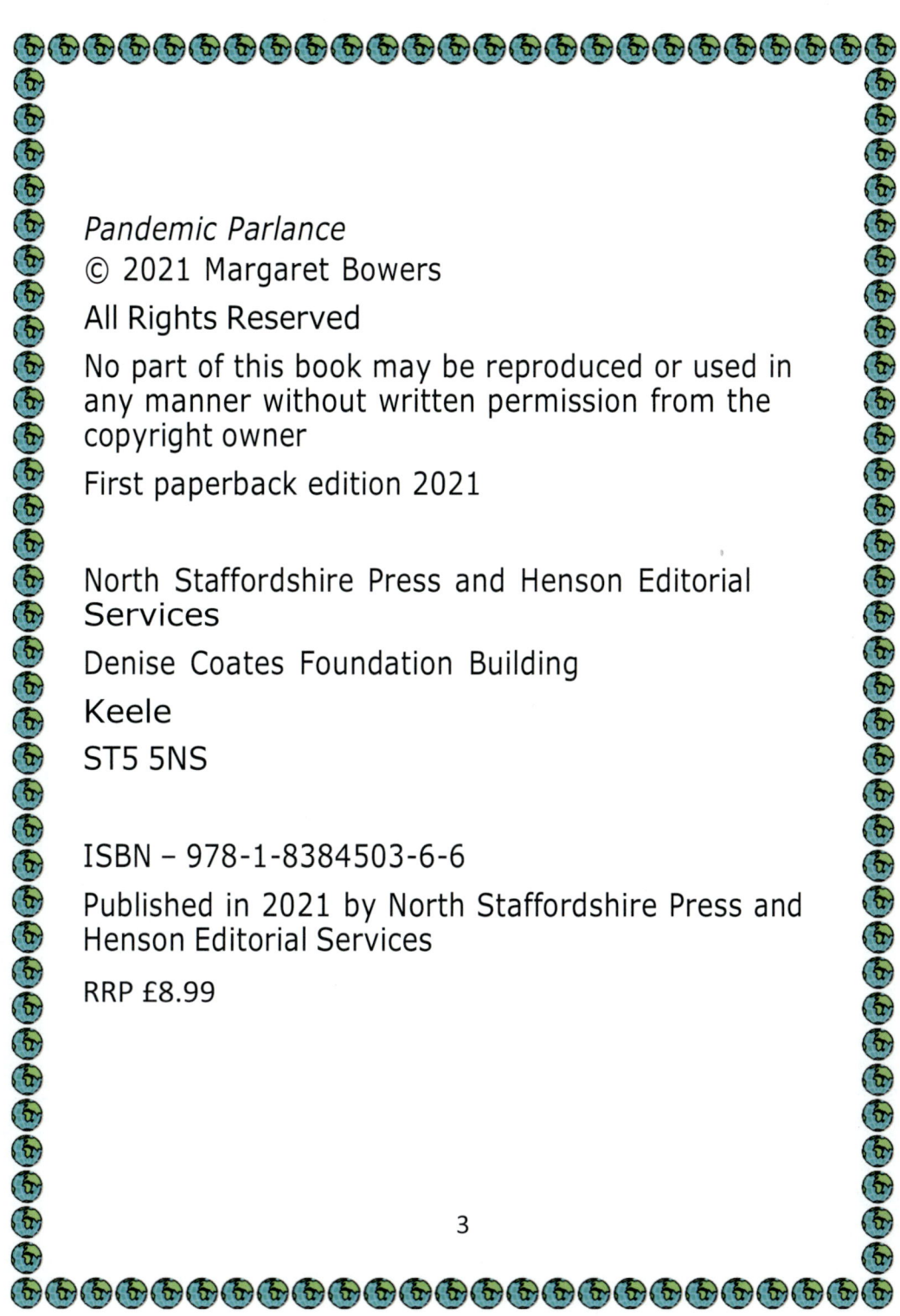

First paperback edition 2021

North Staffordshire Press and Henson Editorial Services

Denise Coates Foundation Building

Keele

ST5 5NS

ISBN – 978-1-8384503-6-6

Published in 2021 by North Staffordshire Press and Henson Editorial Services

RRP £8.99

4

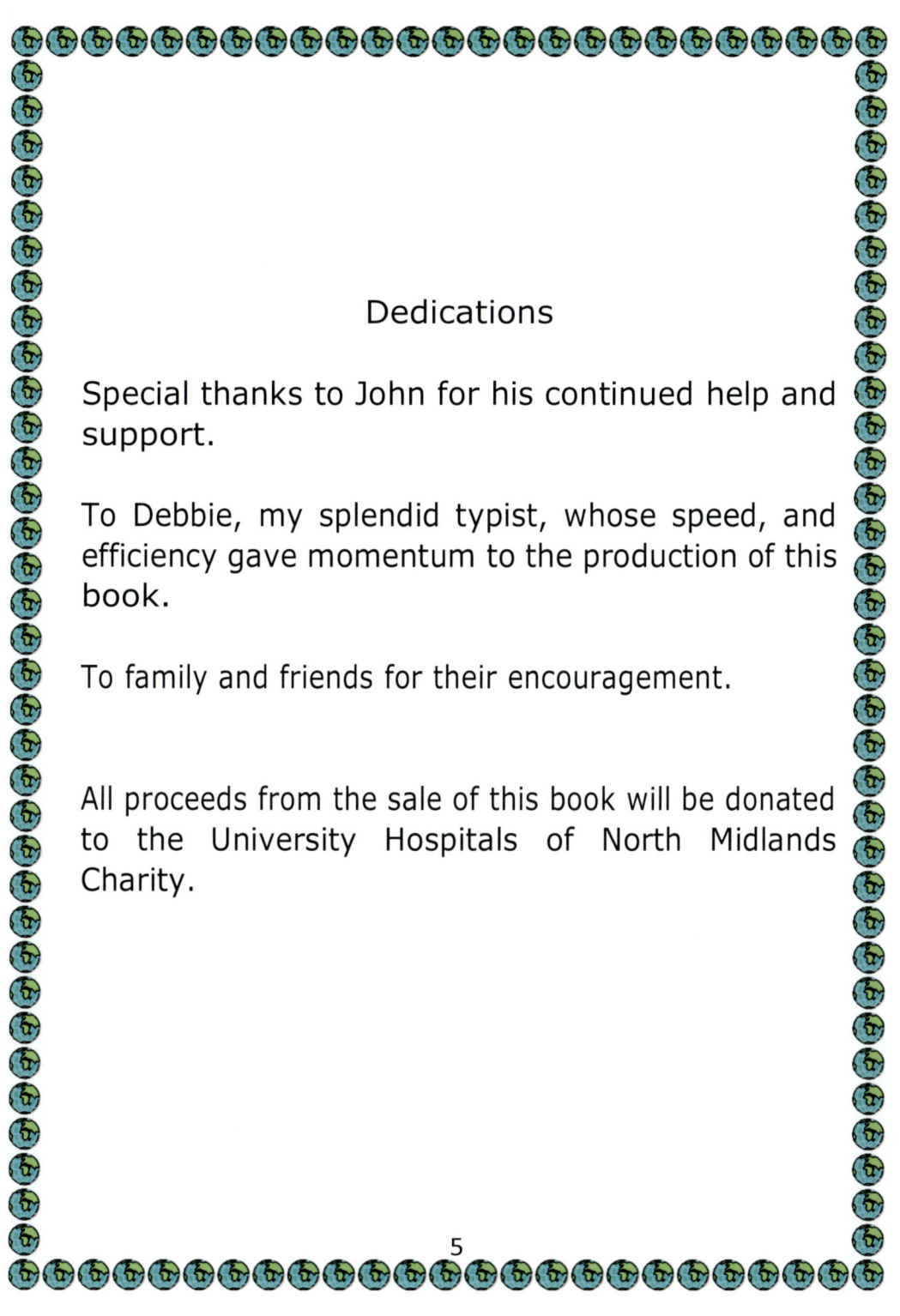

Dedications

Special thanks to John for his continued help and support.

To Debbie, my splendid typist, whose speed, and efficiency gave momentum to the production of this book.

To family and friends for their encouragement.

All proceeds from the sale of this book will be donated to the University Hospitals of North Midlands Charity.

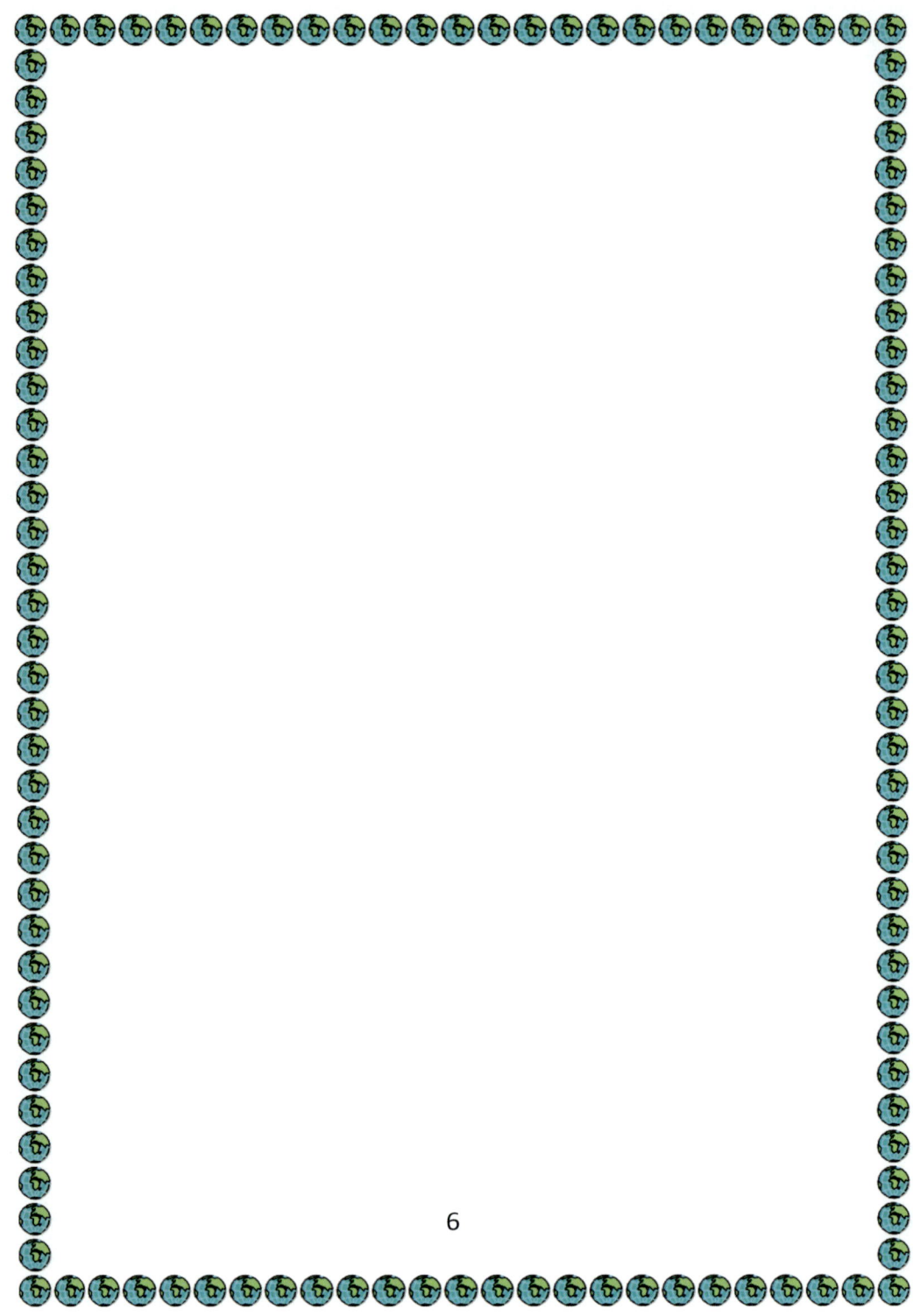

6

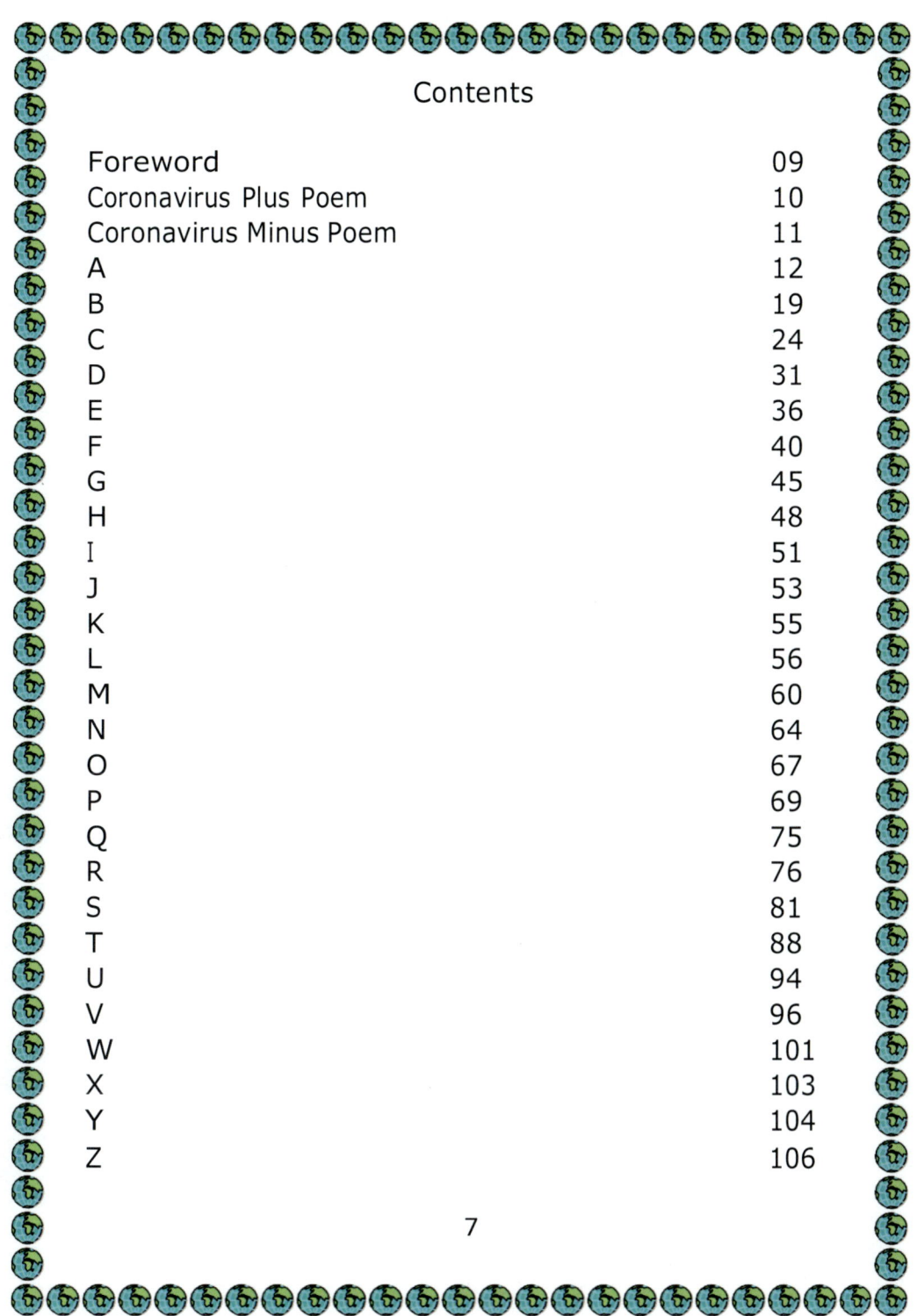

Contents

8

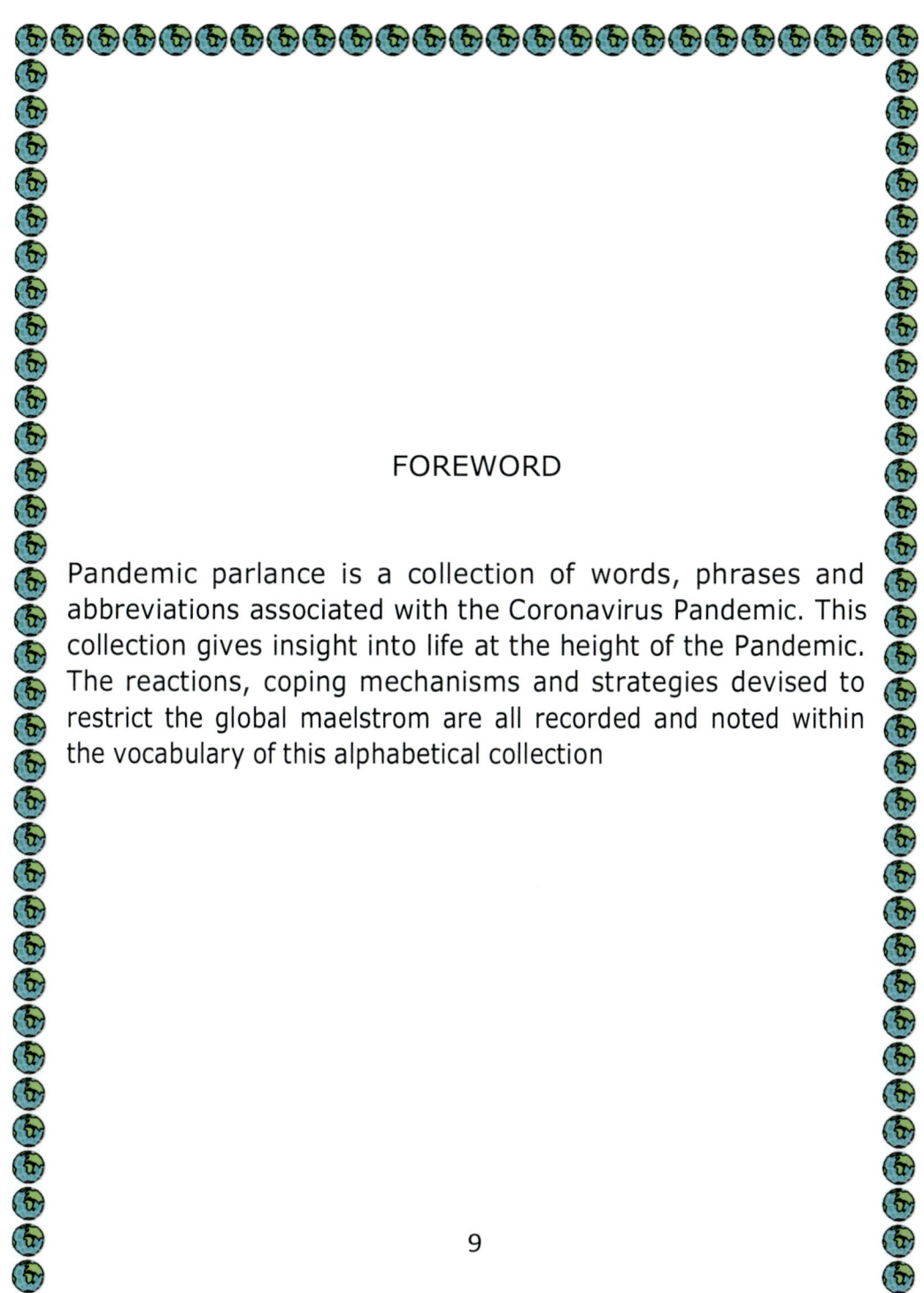

FOREWORD

Pandemic parlance is a collection of words, phrases and abbreviations associated with the Coronavirus Pandemic. This collection gives insight into life at the height of the Pandemic. The reactions, coping mechanisms and strategies devised to restrict the global maelstrom are all recorded and noted within the vocabulary of this alphabetical collection

9

Coronavirus Plus & Minus

PLUS

C   Community caring is firmly in place.

It is proving to be our saving grace.

O   Outstanding front-line workers have excelled during this "Hiatus".

They are now given their due recognition and status.

R   Rationalising the status quo.

Ingenious ways have been devised to soften the blow.

O   Our resilience and adaptability are winning the day.

Realising that things can be done but in a different way.

N   New skills and activities to undertake and learn.

Thereby boosting our self-esteem in turn.

A   Applause and accolades for jobs well done.

Appreciation shown by everyone.

V   Volunteers and Veterans have joined the war.

Their skills are as vital as they were before.

I   Information and intelligence stored on a database.

They will ensure the victory of the human race.

R   Rejoicing that pollution is at an all-time low.

Natural fragrances have an uninhibited flow.

U   Untold simple pleasures, as we exercise, abound.

Blossom trees, exquisite flowers and birds' song has increased in sound.

S   Some lights at the end of the tunnel can be seen.

Namely testing, treatment and Vaccine.

Coronavirus Plus & Minus

MINUS

C   Cut off from family and friend.

      Tactile affirmations of love at an end:

O   Overcome by overwhelming grief and sorrow.

      People wonder how they can face tomorrow.

R   Reality check that 'normal life' is on hold.

      Fighting boredom and depression as the days unfold.

O   Oblivious of the seriousness of the situation.

      Selfish people are a risk to our nation.

N   No school, holidays, or social activity.

      Thereby increasing our feeling of negativity.

A   Aghast at the collateral damage to our education and economy.

      Will we ever regain our autonomy?

V   Various scams have been created.

      Shame on those by whom they were perpetrated.

I   Indifference and ignorance are the enemy.

      If they persist, we will never be free.

R   Retail therapy is no longer available.

      Withdrawal symptoms make us yearn for the unobtainable.

U   Untold suffering too great to endure.

      People unable to take any more.

S   Statistic announcements concerning the virus are diurnal.

      This harrowing pandemic seems eternal.

A

Abuse

During lockdown, the incidences of domestic abuse escalated. Victims were urged to seek help. A code word was given to use on the telephone. Policemen, paramedics, and shop assistants suffered abuse also as people gave vent to their frustration at their restricted lifestyle.

Accident and Emergency Department

People were reluctant to attend these departments for treatment because of their fear of contracting Coronavirus. Safety measures were in place. Areas were cordoned off and colour coded. People were only admitted unaccompanied.

Accolades

Synonyms for the word accolade are praise and approval. Front line workers in the NHS, care sector, public sector, and unsung heroes/ heroines have been singled out, quite deservedly, for accolades in recognition of their fortitude and dedication during this Pandemic.

Adaptability

To be adaptable is to adjust to a new purpose or circumstance. Many businesses have demonstrated their adaptability in ingenious ways. For example – brewers have produced sanitiser, restaurants and cafes have developed their takeaway facility and pubs have sold takeaway cocktails.

Admissions

Hospital admissions, mainly Coronavirus patients, have been at perilous, all-time high. All NHS Staff have coped admirably and tirelessly as the service has approached breaking point.

Advice

Government and medical experts have given advice on a daily basis with regard to a safe course of action to get through the pandemic.

Aftermath

The disastrous effects of this Pandemic will be experienced for countless years to come. Great efforts and ingenuity will be required to cope with the aftermath of the Pandemic. It will be a struggle to resume some sort of normal life, build up the economy and learn to live with the virus which will remain with us.

Ageusia

Loss of taste; A Coronavirus symptom.

Air

During the first lockdown, March 2020, there was hardly any traffic on the road. The air was much fresher and there was less pollution. The natural scents of vegetation and flowers permeated the air.

Air Travel

Air travel ground to a halt. Aeroplanes were parked. Pilots and crew had no work. There was only a minimum number of flights.

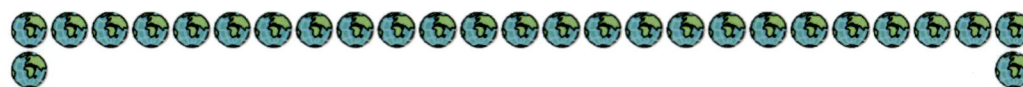

Alert Levels

Alert levels 1-5 gave an indication of the rates of infection increase. Level 5 is the highest rise in infection.

Algorithm

An algorithm is a process or set of rules used in calculation. Because of Coronavirus, examinations were unable to take place. Grades were given on teacher assessments, mock examinations, and algorithm.

Altruism

Altruism is an unselfish concern for or dedication to the interests or welfare of others. People were urged to be altruistic and wear face masks.

Animals

Because of lockdown, towns and villages were deserted. Animals e.g., sheep in Wales became less afraid and timid. They came into towns and villages to forage and explore.

Anosmia

Loss of smell; A Coronavirus symptom.

Antibody

An antibody is a protein produced in the blood to react against the action of a foreign body. It is thought that those who recovered from Coronavirus would have the antibodies.

Anti-Vaccine

A percentage of people have refused to be vaccinated. There have been many anti-vaccine posts on social media. An attempt has been made to remove them.

App

An App is a type of software that allows one to perform specific acts. This software has been used to trace, track, and test those who have been in contact, sometimes unwittingly, with persons infected with Coronavirus.

Applause

Every Thursday at 8pm, people all over the country stepped outside their homes to unite in clapping for the NHS. This was a way of expressing heartfelt appreciation for the brave, tireless and dedicated hard work of all NHS staff.

Appointments

Appointments, for illnesses other than Coronavirus, with consultants and clinical staff were cancelled. The NHS workforce was redeployed to help cope with the overwhelming number of Coronavirus cases.

Appreciation

NHS staff, carers, and frontline workers became aware of an increase in, and recognition of, their value as the nation expressed its gratitude for their work.

Apprenticeships

Because of job losses and businesses closing, the government pledged to introduce meaningful apprenticeships.

17

Astra Zeneca

Astra Zeneca is a drug producing company with headquarters in Cambridge. It was one of the first companies to produce and have a vaccine validated for national use. The Astra Zeneca vaccine is safe, effective and in widespread use to combat Coronavirus.

March / April 2021 – A small number of deaths from Cerebral Venous Sinus Clots (Brain Clots) have been linked with younger people having the vaccine.

Asymptomatic

An asymptomatic person is someone who is infected with the virus but displays no symptoms. The person will, therefore, be unaware that they can infect others.

Austerity

One of the lasting effects of the Pandemic will be economic privation.

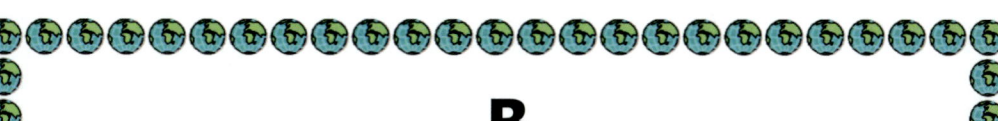

B

Baking

During lockdown many people were baking to pass the time. Baking bread was popular. This led to a shortage of flour in the shops.

Barbecues

Several groups of people were dispersed by the police because they were having illegal barbecues during lockdown. Careless disposal of portable barbecues increased the risk of fires endangering woodlands and heathlands.

Beauty Spots

Beauty spots were declared off limits during lockdown, but crowds thronged to them. Parking at these locations was impossible and illegal.

Behind Closed Doors

Many sporting events e.g., football and cricket took place without spectators. Cardboard cut outs were placed on seats to simulate a crowd. Recorded crowd sounds were used to elicit appropriate responses to the players' actions.

Benefits

An increase in universal credit payments and the furlough scheme were introduced during the first lockdown. £1,000 was given to business owners who kept staff on after furlough ended. These benefits were extended because of subsequent lockdowns.

Bereavements

Families were unable to say goodbye to dying relatives. The number of people attending funerals was limited. The cost of cremations increased.

Bicycles

There were increased sales and use of bicycles. Cars remained parked at home. Lockdown rules only allowed limited travel.

Billions

The government spent billions on projects as a result of the Pandemic e.g., Nightingale hospitals.

Bio Terrorist

This is an extract from an article in the Sunday Mail, 31.05.2020. "Nature has created this virus and has proven once again to be the most effective Bio-Terrorist."

Birds' Song

During lockdown, birds' song could be heard more clearly because there was no traffic noise.

Bookcases

Bookcases have been constant features in the background of Zoom interviews, consultations etc. Some authors have had the blatant audacity to display copies of their book which is subliminal advertising.

Border Control

In 2021, new variants of the virus were discovered in the UK - South African and Brazilian. The presence of new variants resulted in the closing of travel corridors and more stringent border controls. The new variants are purported to be more contagious and deadly.

Boredom

Lockdown and self-isolation meant that people became more creative to alleviate boredom e.g., virtual choirs, keep fit, craft making, cooking, and baking etc.

British Board of Commerce

The British Board of Commerce was asked to cut levies e.g., VAT in order to alleviate poverty.

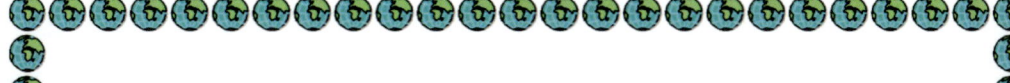

Bubbles

This was the name given to the exclusive, limited groups formed by families or friends for multiple support and socialising in order to combat loneliness and isolation.

Buddy

This was the name given to altruistic people who volunteered to help those without families by shopping and / or collecting medication for them.

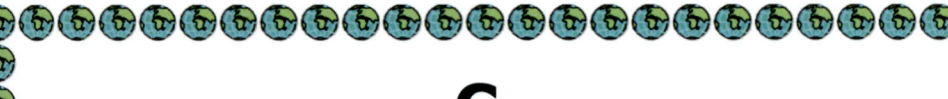

C

Cafes

During the lockdown, cafes were closed. Staff were furloughed. Some income was generated by preparing and selling takeaways. A number of cafes gave free takeaway meals to NHS staff. The meals were delivered to hospitals.

Car Sales

As showrooms were closed, there were reduced numbers of car sales.

Care Homes

Initially, care homes bore the brunt of the virus. Residents were being sent home from hospital without being tested for the virus. Care home staff had no PPE. The virus spread rapidly and there were many avoidable deaths. Some care home staff did not return to their families and homes at the height of the pandemic; they stayed in the care homes to look after the residents. At the time, the state of affairs in care homes was viewed as a scandal and anathema.

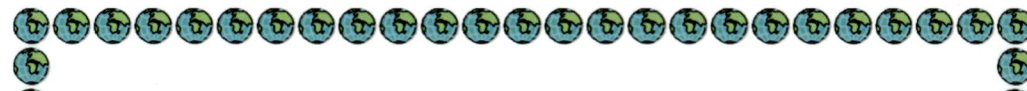

Carers

All carers both in care homes and in the community showed selfless dedication. Home visits continued even though PPE was in short supply.

Charities

Income from fund raising events "fell off a cliff" overnight. All the usual money raising events were postponed indefinitely.

Chiropodists

Chiropodists dealt mainly with emergencies and the vulnerable. They adhered to strict precautionary measures and wore PPE. Hand sanitising and social distancing took place. Waiting rooms were closed. They dealt with fewer clients so that all furniture etc. could be sanitised.

Churches

As churches were closed, "virtual services" took place. Later, churches were opened for short, supervised periods for private prayer.

Circuit Breaker

This was the name given to the time when short, sharp restrictions were imposed to contain or halt the spread of the virus.

Clap For Carers

This demonstration of appreciation took place on 9th July 2020 at 8pm.

Clarity

Clarity is the quality of being clear and easily understood. A synonym is transparency. Clarity is one of the many "BUZZWORDS" used during the Pandemic. It was used whenever the government brought out new measures and coping mechanisms as people tended to interpret them in different ways.

Clots

Blood clots amass in the lungs of those severely ill with Coronavirus. A small number of cases of blood clots, in the brain in particular, have been reported after receiving the Astra Zeneca vaccine.

Cohorts

As the vaccine was rolled out, people were organised into larger groups or cohorts. Members of the cohorts were assembled in order of age (starting with the oldest) and vulnerability.

Community

Community spirit came to the fore during these difficult times.

Compliant

To be compliant is to meet rules or standards. Most people have adhered to lockdown restrictions. There have, however, been some backsliders, particularly during lockdowns 2 and 3.

Consultants

Many consultants have been drafted away from their usual spheres of work to Coronavirus duties.

Consultations

Consultations with doctors and consultants were conducted, in the main, by telephone.

Councils

Councils have had difficulty dealing with the aftermath of the Pandemic due to a shortage of money.

Coronavirus (COVID-19)

Coronavirus / Covid 19 is thought to have started from an animal market in China. It is a ZOONOTIC virus i.e., a virus that jumps from animals to humans.

Corridors

Corridors of Travel, between reciprocal countries that did not require self-isolation before and after visiting, were set up. These corridors existed until new variants of the virus emerged forcing tighter border controls.

Cough

A persistent cough is a Coronavirus symptom.

Courts

A huge backlog of cases built up. This resulted in criminals getting lesser sentences and the setting up of Nightingale courts.

COVID Code

This is a code, similar to the Highway Code. It gives rules, regulations, and requirements to which everyone must adhere in order to get through the Pandemic safely.

Crime

The number of criminal cases decreased but other crimes e.g., scams, were perpetuated. The scams were mainly in connection with Coronavirus.

D

Day Trippers

In spite of the restrictions and limitations on travel, hundreds of people flocked to the beaches (Bournemouth in particular) and beauty spots. There was illegal parking. At the end of the day, there was a disgusting amount of litter left behind.

Death Rate

Daily announcements were made about the number of people who had died from Coronavirus. Great Britain was ranked amongst the European countries with a high death rate. It is interesting to note that no deaths from Influenza were recorded in 2020. Also, letters appeared in newspapers from people saying that their relatives had not died from Coronavirus but, because the virus was a contributing factor listed on the death certificate, they were counted among the Coronavirus death rate statistics.

Deliveries

Delivery companies were kept extremely busy as food, clothes, household goods etc, were all ordered online.

Demacian

On his show, Andrew Marr said that a "Demacian attitude" was needed to get through this Pandemic. The people of Demacia were fiercely proud. They had a prestigious military history. In their strong, lawful society, ideals of justice, honour and duty were highly valued.

Dentists

Initially, dentists dealt mainly with emergencies. Access to the dentist was via a telephone conversation with a triage dental nurse. Within the dental practice strict precautionary measures were in place.

Depression

Lockdown, self-isolation, and lack of contact with loved ones caused many people to suffer from depression.

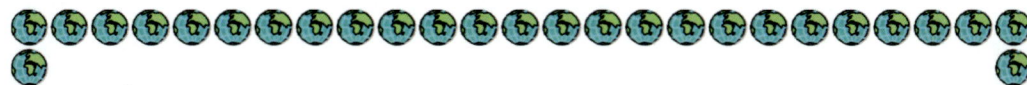

Detail

New Coronavirus guidelines and protocols had to be studied in detail because "The Devil's in the detail".

Dexamethasone

Dexamethasone is a cheap, effective treatment in some cases for Coronavirus. It is a steroid which has been in use since the 1960s.

Disadvantaged

The following groups were disadvantaged during the Pandemic:
1. Families trying to home school without a computer. The situation was eased when the general public responded quite generously to appeals to donate their old computers/laptops/tablets.
2. Those with limited income.
3. People with disabilities, such as the deaf, were unable to lip read due to masks being worn.

Disruption

Everything such as weddings, holidays, celebrations, and education were "on hold".

Distancing

One of the safety measures was social distancing. Everyone was urged to keep 2 metres apart.

Divide

Social and educational divides will be manifested as a result of the Pandemic.

Doctors

Access to surgeries and face to face consultations with doctors was limited. Consultations were by telephone in the main.

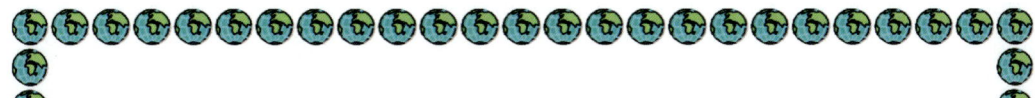

Dog Walking

During lockdown, dog walking was a form of allowed exercise. Many dogs had been purchased with no thought for their welfare when work resumed.

E

Ease

Compliance with lockdown rules meant that restrictions became less severe. They were lifted gradually and carefully. Lockdown easing was keenly anticipated.

Ebola

Drugs used during the Ebola epidemic have been tried in the treatment of Coronavirus. They have been effective in some cases.

Economy

Economy encompasses the state of a country in terms of its production and consumption of goods and services and the supply of money. The Pandemic caused great economic uncertainty. Businesses were unable to operate. Staff were laid off or furloughed. The young were affected in particular.

Education

Schools were closed to all pupils with the exception of children of front-line workers and those at risk. Parents were home schooling with the assistance of work set by teachers online and activity programmes on the television. Schools re-opened after the first lockdown but closed again because of rising infection rates. After a third lockdown, the re-opening of schools on March 8th, 2021, was a priority. Strict guidelines were in place. Older pupils were taught to use lateral flow tests for signs of the virus.

Efficacy

Efficacy was the word used in connection with the roll out of the vaccine and also about the vaccine itself.

Epidemiology

This is the title of the sphere of medicine dealing with epidemic diseases.

Essential

At the height of the Pandemic, during lockdown, shopping was only allowed for essential items. Journeys were restricted to essential travel.

Examinations

Examinations 2020 were disrupted and unable to take place. Grades were awarded on the following criteria:

1. Teacher Assessments
2. Mock examinations
3. An Algorithm (Process or set of rules used in calculations)

Consequently, many pupils were downgraded causing great distress and scathing criticism of the government. This method of awarding grades was called "The Triple Lock System". Parents and children could appeal the results. Pupils also had the option to re-sit examinations Autumn 2020. However, after much disquiet, greater emphasis was placed on teacher assessments. Pupils received upgraded results. In 2021, disruption of examinations remained unavoidable. Grades will be awarded by teacher assessment, taking into account course work and mock examinations.

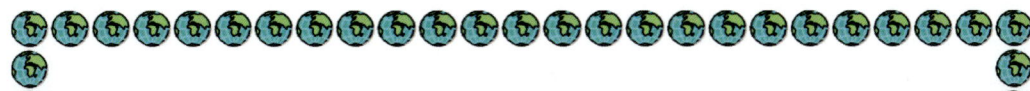

Exercise

Exercise was essential during lockdown. During the first lockdown, over 70s were allowed 1 hour per day local exercise. Other age groups were included in consequent lockdowns.

Exponential

This adjective is used when describing something becoming more and more rapid. It indicates an increase. The adverb exponentially is my "word of the Pandemic". It was used on a daily basis.

F

Face Masks

Expert opinions were divided initially over the effectiveness of face masks. Now, they are regarded as an essential element of the "Package of Safety Measures". At first, face masks were only mandatory on public transport, now their use is required and widespread. A variety of masks are available. Some are single use; others are multiple use but must be washed at 60 degrees. Masks must be put on, removed, and disposed of in a particular way to ensure their effectiveness and reduce the transmission of the virus.

Fake News

Fake news led to scaremongering and panic buying resulting in a shortage of products in shops and supermarkets.

Finances

The management and supply of money was in turmoil. Many businesses have seen their financial resources drained and a number have ceased trading. Businesses and people have had to rely on government financial support.

Firebreak

An area or areas have been put in lockdown for a designated period of time e.g., 16 days hoping that this will act like a "Firebreak" to stop the spread of the virus.

Flour

During lockdown, baking became increasingly popular, particularly the production of bread. This led to a shortage of flour.

Food Banks

Food banks have been vital resources and lifelines. They have been busier than ever. People have been generous with their donations and have volunteered to help with distribution to those who are housebound.

Formula One

Breathing apparatus, used by Formula One drivers, was modified to help overcome the shortage of ventilators in hospitals.

Freedom

This has been curtailed and restricted in all spheres and walks of life. People have been required to comply with restrictions in order to reduce the spread of the virus.

Free Meal Vouchers

Free meal vouchers were issued solely for use in term-time, but Marcus Rashford (a footballer with Manchester United and England) has campaigned successfully for them to be supplied in the school holidays.

Front Line Workers

Front line workers include:
1. ALL NHS WORKERS
2. CARE WORKERS

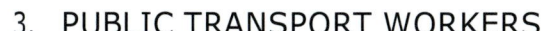

3. PUBLIC TRANSPORT WORKERS
4. REFUSE COLLECTORS
5. SOCIAL WORKERS
6. TEACHERS IN SCHOOLS FOR FRONTLINE WORKERS' CHILDREN
7. SHOP ASSISTANTS (PARTICULARLY SUPERMARKETS)
8. CHEMISTS

Funding

The Government has been called upon to fund projects and keep businesses viable.

Fund Raising

With the advent of lockdown, fund raising events came to a halt and many charities had no sources of income to carry on their vital work. Individuals and groups performed outstanding feats in order to raise money for good causes e.g., CAPTAIN SIR TOM MOORE raised well over 30 million pounds for the NHS by completing 100 lengths in his garden with the aid of a walker. There have been many men, women and children who have performed feats of endurance to raise money.

Funerals

The number of mourners permitted to attend funerals was limited.

Furlough

Originally, furlough was a military term. Personnel were granted leave of absence from duty. This term was used during the Pandemic for staff who were given permission to be away from their work and a percentage of their pay was funded by the government. Furlough was extended through all lockdowns.

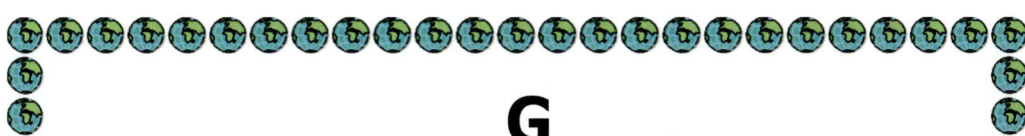

G

Gardens

During lockdown, those who had gardens found them a boon. Plants and trees seemed to flourish. Their scents filled the air because of lack of traffic pollution.

Garden Centres

Lockdown restrictions meant that garden centres were closed for crucial months but then they were allowed to re-open under strict social distancing rules.

GDP

Gross Domestic Product is the final value of the goods and services produced within the geographical boundaries of a country during a specified period of time – normally a year. GDP growth rate is an important indicator of the economic performance of a country.

Generosity

People have been extremely generous in these difficult times freely giving time, help, money and food.

Genetic Code (of the virus)

The numbers of the virus which give an indication of how the virus is evolving and mutating.

Genome

Information about the composition of the virus.

Goodwill

Everyone was caring for and about each other and wishing them well.

Government

The government, with the advice of the experts, had to make decisions concerning unprecedented conditions. A "bottomless money box" has been needed.

Grief

To their immense sorrow, people were not allowed to be with their dying loved ones. Numbers at funerals were limited.

Guidance

The government issued guidance on a regular basis (daily, weekly, monthly etc.) to help cope with the Pandemic.

Gyms

Gyms were closed for months but later re-opened under strict guidelines. People took green exercise (i.e., they exercised in parks and beauty spots).

H

Hairdressers

During the first lockdown, hairdressers were closed for 3 months. When they re-opened, it was under strict social distancing rules. On entry to the salon, temperatures were taken and hands sanitised. The hairdressers wore PPE and partitions were placed between sinks and mirrors. All furniture and equipment was sanitised after each client. Once again during the third lockdown, hairdressers were closed. They re-opened on April 12th, 2021.

Hardship

The Pandemic has caused untold hardship. In his summer statement (08.07.2020) the Chancellor of the Exchequer, Rishi Sunak, said, "Hardship lies ahead".

Herd Immunity

At least 60% of the population needs to be vaccinated in order to achieve herd immunity. When achieved, it will mean that the virus cannot be spread and transmitted so easily.

Heterologist Vaccination

This vaccine is the result of mixing doses from different vaccines.

Hidden Gems

During lockdown, people reconnected with nature and rediscovered local beauty spots / hidden gems.

Holidays

Many holidays abroad were cancelled, and people took "staycations" or holidays at home. When restrictions were reduced, there was a sharp rise in Coronavirus cases in some countries. On returning from these countries, strict quarantine rules were imposed i.e.,14 days self-isolation. These countries reciprocated and insisted on isolation for 14 days on arrival.

"Holiday Hunger"

Holiday hunger was experienced by children who were eligible for free school meals. However, these meals were not available during the school holidays. A campaign led by the footballer Marcus Rashford was successful in eradicating this hardship.

(SEE FREE MEAL VOUCHERS, HOME SCHOOLING AND EDUCATION)

Hospitals

At the height of the first wave of the Pandemic (and subsequent waves), hospitals were approaching capacity. Initially, PPE was in short supply. Emergency hospitals were constructed. (SEE NIGHTINGALE HOSPITALS)

Hotels

There were few occupants in hotels. The government paid some hotels to give shelter to the homeless. This meant that there were fewer people sleeping rough on the streets.

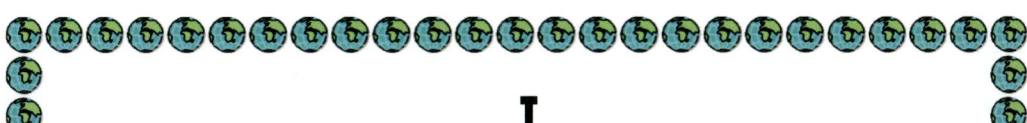

I

Inconsiderate

On the whole, people were kind and community spirited. Some people (in a minority) were inconsiderate, flouting safety procedures and protocol.

Infection Surveys

Infection surveys have been carried out by The National Institute for Health Protection (NIHP) to monitor the spread of the virus and help with preventative measures e.g., local lockdowns.

Intensive Care

In the early stages, and subsequent waves of the Pandemic, the intensive care wards were overwhelmed by the number of patients requiring specialist treatment.

International Travel – Traffic Light System

This system was introduced prior to international travel being allowed to take place. Countries were colour coded according to their infection levels. Red indicated high Covid levels. Travellers had to self-isolate in a hotel on returning to the UK. Yellow indicated medium Covid levels. Anyone returning to the UK from a country with a yellow code had to self-isolate at home. Countries with a green code did not warrant any self-isolation. Tests prior to departure and on arrival were mandatory for all colour codes.

Intubate

An incision is made in the throat so that ventilator tubes can be inserted.

Isolation

Many people, especially those with serious conditions, had to self-isolate for long periods of time. Also, anyone who had been in contact with someone diagnosed with Coronavirus had to self-isolate for 14 days. Those returning from overseas holidays in a county with a high infection rate had to self-isolate for 14 days or be fined.

J

Jargon

Many specialized or technical words and terms, mainly of a scientific nature, were used and introduced during the Pandemic.

JCVI

Joint Committee on Vaccination and Immunisation.

Jogging

Jogging was an increasingly popular pastime during lockdown.

Johnson (Boris, Prime Minister UK)

In the early stages of the Pandemic, Boris Johnson, the UK Prime Minister, succumbed to the virus. He was treated in St Thomas's hospital, London and was discharged April 12th, 2020.

JSS (Job Support Scheme)

This was a government initiative to replace furlough which was due to end October 2020. Through the JSS scheme, eligible claimants would get 2/3 of their salary. However, the furlough scheme was extended.

K

Kindness

The Pandemic brought out the best in people. There were many acts of a caring, considerate, benevolent, selfless, public spirited and altruistic nature.

L

Landlords

Landlords were asked to be understanding when people had difficulty paying their rents regularly, particularly student lets. The government intervened to lengthen the time before eviction would take place.

Laptops

There was a shortage of availability of laptops for home schooling. Disadvantaged families were affected most. Public appeals on television resulted in generous donations of used laptops, tablets etc. These were cleaned of their data then distributed to those in need.

Lateral Flow Tests

These tests are in general use for the public and pupils in particular. Results are given in 30 minutes. People who are asymptomatic are revealed. Positive lateral flow tests had results confirmed by a laboratory test.

Learning Disabilities

Those with learning disabilities had a difficult time because, due to the Pandemic, help was not readily available. The wearing of face masks compounded difficulties. For instance, those who are deaf found it difficult to lip read.

Life Chances

There is great concern that children have missed so much time in school that they are way behind with abilities and knowledge. Their life chances i.e., employment expertise etc. will be seriously damaged.

Light Pollution

During the Pandemic and lockdown restrictions there was less light pollution. This meant that the celestial wonders of the night sky could be seen in all their glory. Nocturnal creatures such as bats have benefited also.

Litter

An increasing and inordinate amount of litter was left in parks and beauty spots costing time and money to clear.

Lockdown

Lockdown was originally a prison term used when prisoners were locked in their cells for long periods of time. The whole country was placed in lockdown for two months initially. Later on, there were isolated lockdowns as cases of Coronavirus grew in certain areas (e.g., Leicester). Further national lockdowns ensued.

Long Covid

After recovering from Covid,, there are some long-term effects such as: -
PHYSICAL –Difficulty in breathing, tiredness, and lack of energy.
MENTAL –Depression, memory loss etc.

Lungs

Coronavirus causes scaring of the lungs, fluid on the lungs and clots. (SEE VENTILATORS)

M

Mandatory

Adjectives derived from the noun mandate are order and command. During the Pandemic, many of the restrictions were mandatory. They were put in place to halt the spread of the virus.

Markets

Open air markets have been allowed to trade. It is thought that the Pandemic does not spread as easily in the open air with social distancing.

Masks

See "F" – Face Masks

MHRA

This stands for the Medicines and Healthcare products Regulatory Agency. This agency assess data recorded when new products have been tried before they can be "rolled out" to the general public. Its aim is to ensure pharmacological excellence through vigilance.

Mental Health

Mental health problems increased during lockdown and the restrictions imposed in an attempt curb the spread of the virus. People were isolated, lonely, afraid, and desperate to see their family and friends.

Metres

Social distancing mandates that people must keep 2 metres apart. This was changed later to 1 + metres but 2 metres is still advocated.

Midwives

Midwives have been busy and hardworking as usual. Life (and death) goes on.

Milkmen

Lockdown and restrictions saw a return to doorstop deliveries, not only of milk but of bread and groceries. It was a time of "Renaissance" for milkmen.

Minks

Millions of minks have had to be culled in Denmark because they were found to be carrying a mutated form of the virus. Two hundred workers have been affected. If the mutated version of the virus had spread, it could have nullified the work done to find a vaccine.

Misinformation

As this is an unprecedented, new "infant" virus, there have been false rumours and claims concerning it. Scaremongering has been rife.

Monoclonal Antibodies

Scientists have made the following discovery about antibodies: There are two antibodies which attach themselves to the Coronavirus spike, if one fails, the other takes over.

Mortgage "Holidays"

Some mortgage payments were suspended during lockdown.

Motorists

Lockdown meant that there was less traffic on the roads. Some motorists behaved irresponsibly and flouted speed restrictions.

Mutate

Just as the Influenza virus changes and alters on a regular basis, it is thought that this could be the case with Coronavirus.

N

NIHP

National Institute for Health Protection (SEE INFECTION SURVEY).

Negative Influences

The negative influences of Covid safety measures are manifold:

1. Face masks present difficulties for the deaf and visually impaired.
2. Difficulties experienced by disabled people have been compounded.
3. There were catastrophic effects on the economy and livelihoods.
4. Mental distress has been caused.

NERVTAG

New and Emerging Respiratory Virus Threats Advisory Group.

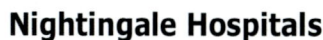

Nightingale Hospitals

The year 2020 was the 200th year since the birth of Florence Nightingale. There was a "Shine a Light" celebration. Nightingale hospitals were constructed in some cities to treat the great number of Coronavirus patients as wards in hospitals were reaching capacity. Fortunately, they were not needed, and some have been put to other uses e.g., treating patients with illnesses and incapacities other than Coronavirus.

Non-Essential Businesses

These businesses include some shops, car showrooms etc. All were closed during lockdown.

Normality

Getting our lives back "to normal" was on everyone's wish list.

Nurses

Nurses, along with all NHS workers were appreciated greatly. They received many plaudits and accolades. Some nurses and doctors came out of retirement to help. There was a great recruitment drive, and many came forward and expressed an interest in joining the NHS. (SEE ALSO CLAP FOR THE NHS AND CLAP FOR CARERS)

O

Oesophagus

Ventilator breathing tubes were inserted into the oesophagus of seriously ill patients.

ONS

Office for National Statistics. Their numbers for Coronavirus deaths were considerably higher than those published daily. (SEE INFECTION SURVEY)

On Hold

Many events e.g., holidays, weddings, birthday celebrations etc. were postponed and kept "on hold" because of the Pandemic.

Opticians

Opticians' premises were closed during lockdown. When restrictions were lifted, they opened following government guidelines and procedures.

Oxygen

Coronavirus causes breathing difficulties. Oxygen was given, in some cases via the oesophagus.

P

Pandemic

Pandemic is a Greek word meaning "people all around the world". A universal epidemic, Coronavirus is worldwide.

Parks

Parks were used constantly for exercise and enjoyment of plants, trees, lakes, birds on water and in trees. (SEE PLAYGROUNDS)

Pasta

A fear that food might be in short supply resulted in bulk buying of pasta by some people. The concerns proved to be unfounded.

Pathogen

A pathogen is a micro-organism or agent that causes disease. ADJECTIVE –Pathogenic.

Payrolls

Some businesses failed during lockdown. People lost their jobs and instead of being on a payroll were on benefits.

PCR Test

Stands for Polymerase Chain Reaction Test. It is a diagnostic test to determine infection by analysing a sample to see if it contains genetic material from the virus.

Persistent

A persistent cough is one of the symptoms of Coronavirus.

Picnics

Coronavirus is not thought to be passed from person to person so easily in the open air. Many people took advantage of the good weather post lockdown restrictions to have picnics.

PICS

Post Intensive Care Syndrome. Coronavirus left many patients with aftereffects such as: - breathing difficulty, fatigue, mental problems etc.

Pinch Points

Areas where it is difficult to social distance.

Playgrounds

During lockdown, children's playgrounds were closed. When restrictions were lifted, they were opened but national guidelines had to be observed.

Pollution

During lockdown there was hardly any traffic on the road, therefore less fumes and pollution. The sky seemed bluer. Everywhere and everything looked brighter. The scent of flowers and blossoms filled the air.

Postponement

Many events – weddings, birthday parties, holidays and all manner of celebrations had to be postponed.

PPE

Personal Protective Equipment. This was in short supply at the height of the first wave of the Pandemic. Some PPE was sourced from abroad. People made PPE to help the NHS.

Pregnant Ladies

Pregnant ladies are particularly vulnerable to the virus at 28 weeks.

Prison Officers

Social distancing proved problematic, especially when escorting handcuffed prisoners. Lockdown is a prison term. (SEE LOCKDOWN)

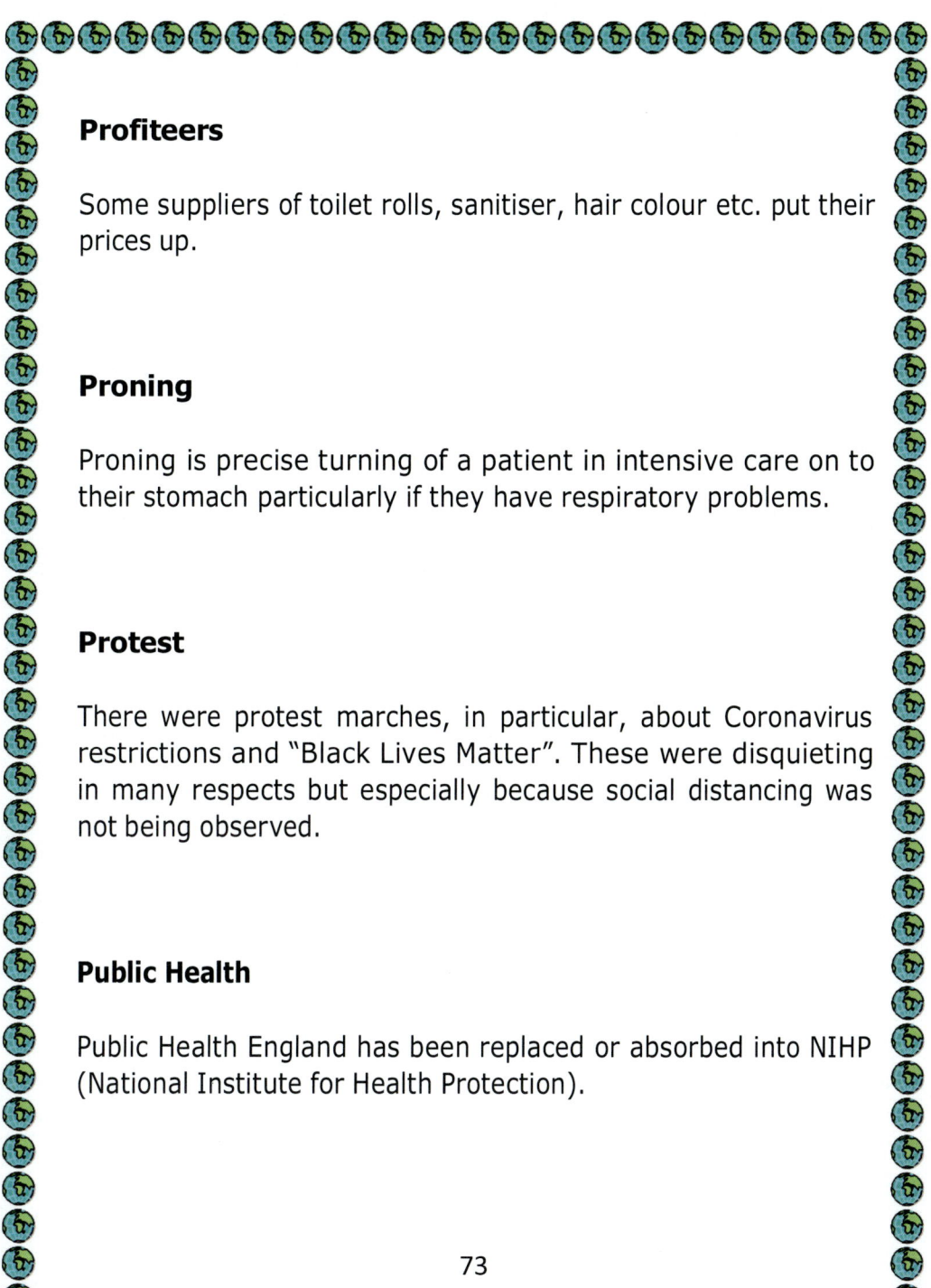

Profiteers

Some suppliers of toilet rolls, sanitiser, hair colour etc. put their prices up.

Proning

Proning is precise turning of a patient in intensive care on to their stomach particularly if they have respiratory problems.

Protest

There were protest marches, in particular, about Coronavirus restrictions and "Black Lives Matter". These were disquieting in many respects but especially because social distancing was not being observed.

Public Health

Public Health England has been replaced or absorbed into NIHP (National Institute for Health Protection).

Public Toilets

Councils had already closed a large number of public toilets. The remaining toilets were closed during lockdown causing difficulties for the disabled and those with bladder and bowel problems. It also impacted those out exercising.

Public Transport

Buses, trains, and taxis were virtually empty. The wearing of face masks in these vehicles was mandatory.

PVS

Post Viral Syndrome. (SEE PICS)

Q

Quarantine

The word Quarantine originates from Venice. Sailors, returning to Venice after voyages with diseases had to stay offshore for 40 days. Quaranta is Italian for 40.

Queen's Speeches

The Queen has made two broadcasts to the nation during these troubled times.

Questions

There were many questions demanding clarity after new restrictions were imposed.

Queueing

Queues formed outside shops and supermarkets. People were allowed to enter providing social distancing could be observed.

R

"R" Number

The "R" number or Reproduction number is an indication of the virulence of the virus. 1 is the significant number. If the R number is below 1, the spread of the virus is contained. Above 1 indicates a rise in the number of people who will be infected.

Rainbow

Pictures of rainbows were made (especially by children) and displayed on windows. Some were displayed on walls, in fields etc. The pictures of rainbows were to show solidarity and support for the NHS.

Ramp Up

This means to increase effort and therefore output, many initiatives such as testing, and vaccination were ramped up.

Rapid

Rapid/speedy test results were optimal.

Recession

Recession is a time when trade and industrial activity are reduced.

Reconnect

During lockdown when travel was restricted or forbidden, many people visited local beauty sports or discovered new ones; they reconnected with nature.

Redundancy

Redundancy was at an all time high (324,000 July - Sept 2020). Many were made redundant prior to furlough ending but then it was extended to March 2021.

Rent Rebates

Many students were eligible for rent rebates during lockdown, but they had difficulty obtaining them.

Resilience

Resilience is the ability to cope with, withstand, adapt, or recover from difficult conditions. Resilience was in evidence during the Pandemic.

Results

Rapid results from testing and tracing were a powerful tool in keeping the Pandemic in check.

Rights

People's rights are an important consideration when imposing any restrictions.

Risk Assessment

During these unprecedented times, risk assessment was of paramount importance to ensure everyone's safety during any activities.

RNLI

The sterling work of the RNLI was in evidence, in a limited capacity, during lockdown.

Roll Out

Information and ways forward were rolled out initially on a daily basis.

Rough Sleepers

Many rough sleepers were taken off the streets and accommodated in hotels.

Royal Family

Prince Charles fell victim to Coronavirus. Also, Prince William was infected but his illness at the time was not put into the public domain.

S

SAGE

This is the Scientific Advisory Group for Emergencies i.e. The government's scientific advisory body. Advice was given on all things to do with Coronavirus.

Sanitiser

Widely available and used to sanitise hands when entering all types of buildings - shops, hospitals, doctors' surgeries etc.

Scams

Some unscrupulous individuals took advantage of these unprecedented times to perpetrate scams of all types.

Scaring

Coronavirus has left scaring of the lungs and breathing difficulties.

Schools

Most schools were closed during lockdown except for access by children of frontline workers and vulnerable children. Home schooling was employed using computers to access work supplied by teachers. Learning programmes were designed to be followed online. After lockdown, government guidelines were followed to put safety measures in place so that schools could re-open safely. Children are not affected as badly or seriously by the virus, although they could infect relatives. The importance of schooling meant that keeping schools open was a priority. The loss of education is detrimental to our nations' future place in the world.

Scrubs (SEE PPE)

The clothing worn by hospital personnel. When this became in short supply, many people made it for the hospital staff.

Self-Isolation

People who contracted Coronavirus had to self-isolate for 14 days. The same procedure applied to people who had been in contact with those who had Coronavirus.

Separation Anxiety

There were concerns that pets (mainly dogs) would become anxious when owners resumed work as they have had constant company.

Shielding

The most vulnerable in society i.e., those with life threatening illnesses, disabilities etc. were advised by letters from the government to self-isolate for 12 weeks initially.

Signs

Sign writers were extremely busy producing signs to reiterate government guidelines for display in public places – streets, parks, hospitals, schools etc.

Smize

A smize is a smile with your eyes when wearing a mask.

Social Distancing

One of the government's guidelines to help halt the spread of the virus. People were recommended to keep 2 metres apart.

Socio-Economic

The Pandemic has had widespread ramifications for social and economic aspects of all countries.

Sorrow

It has been a time of great sorrow for those who have lost loved ones, particularly as it was not possible for relatives to be present at their last moments. Also, numbers at funerals were limited.

Speed Limits

During the first lockdown there was not much traffic on the roads. Faced with empty roads some drivers ignored speed limits.

Spike

When the virus rose to high levels this was called a spike in the Pandemic - a high point.

Spike Protein

The spike protein on the surface of the virus is built by part of the virus's genetic code. It is an essential and vital part of how the vaccine is produced.

Statistics

Facts and data concerning all things pertinent to the virus have been obtained and disseminated from the study of statistics namely the collection and analysis of information shown in numbers.

Strategy / Stratagem

Numerous strategies have had to be planned and carried out in order to limit the effects socially, economically, and politically of the new unseen enemy – The virus.

Subliminal Advertising (SEE BOOKCASES)

Subsidies

Subsidies were given to people and businesses by the government during lockdown and beyond to support them when businesses had to close. Even after lockdown, businesses did not recover because of restrictions and guidelines.

Summer Statement / Budget

The Chancellor of the Exchequer, Rishi Sunak, gave a summer budget statement in view of the stringent economic constraints brought about by these unprecedented times.

Supermarkets

These were, and still are, the mainstay of supplies. They arranged special opening times e.g., for NHS workers, the elderly and disabled to ensure that everyone could shop safely. Sanitiser for hands and trolleys was supplied. Floors were marked out with directional arrows and 2 metre spacing marks.

Support / Social Bubble (SEE BUBBLES)

Symptoms

A list of symptoms to look out for to indicate if one has contracted the virus namely:

1. High temperature
2. Persistent cough
3. Loss of sense of smell (Anosmia)
4. Loss of sense of taste (Ageusia)
5. Lethargy
6. Difficulty breathing

T

Teachers

All schools were closed during the first lockdown except for children of frontline workers and vulnerable children. Scientists said that transmission of the virus among children was low. Staff had to prepare schools for re-opening with safety measures advocated by the government guidelines i.e., sanitising, safe distancing, and masks. With the second lockdown, the government was adamant that schools should remain open, but the spread of the virus was rife, and schools had to close again.

Telephone Consultations

Attendance at hospitals and doctors' surgeries was kept to a minimum. Patients were given telephone consultations. Appropriate action was taken if the information obtained during the telephone consultation deemed it necessary e.g., face to face consultation with a doctor.

Temperature

High temperature is one of the symptoms of Coronavirus. Most establishments took people's temperature before allowing entry. This was often not very accurate.

Testing

The government tried to implement a testing regime in order to combat the spread of the virus. Initially this proved problematic and unsuccessful for a number of reasons: logistics, slow results, people's reluctance to come forward or be contacted (SEE LATERAL FLOW TESTING)

Thank You Day

July 4th, 2021 has been suggested as a 'National Thank You Day' when everyone can express their thanks to all those who have worked tirelessly and selflessly throughout the Pandemic.

Tinned Tomatoes

For some reason tinned tomatoes were in short supply during the first lockdown.

Toilets (SEE PUBLIC TOILETS)

Toilet Rolls

An unfounded rumour that these would be in short supply caused people to panic buy in bulk, leaving empty shelves in many supermarkets. Some supermarkets introduced rationing of these products.

Tracing

Part of the test, track, and trace system. Those who tested positive had their most recent contacts tracked and traced. Apps were displayed at the entrance to venues for signing in.

Tracking (SEE TESTING AND TRACING)

Traffic Light System

In order to attempt to avoid another national lockdown, the government introduced a three-tier system. Areas were categorised into the coloured system according to the number of cases in a particular region i.e., green – medium, yellow – high, red – very high. Restrictions were most severe in those areas placed in the red category where the Pandemic was most virulent. A fourth even more restrictive tier was introduced Oct. / Nov. 2020. The next step would be lockdown.

Trains

Masks were mandatory on stations and in trains. Trains were not widely used.

Transfers

At the height of the first wave of the Pandemic, intensive care wards at some hospitals had reached capacity. Patients were transferred in specially equipped ambulances with highly trained staff to other hospitals where beds were available. Transfer journeys undertaken were, in some cases, as far as 200 to 300 miles away.

Transmission

An indication of the rate of transmission of the virus is given by the "R" number or reproduction number.

Transparency

This word was in evidence whenever new restrictions were introduced. People wanted to know the justification for them.

Treatment

As the virus became more prevalent hospitals found different drugs and treatments to be effective.

Triple lock appeal system (SEE EXAMINATIONS)

Trump (President Donald)

President Donald Trump succumbed to the virus but made quite a speedy recovery.

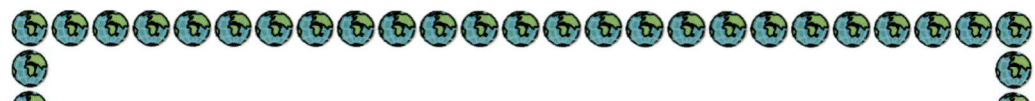

Trust

Owing to the unprecedented nature of the Pandemic people had to put a lot of trust in scientists, experts, and NHS staff.

Tube Trains

The crowding on the tube in London was very concerning in the early days of the Pandemic as there was no social distancing.

U

Unemployment

The Pandemic has resulted in higher levels of unemployment. During restrictions and lockdown, many businesses were unable to trade and closed. Some staff were put on furlough, but others lost their jobs. It was difficult to find employment. Many staff decided to re-train.

Unions

As always, unions were there to support members but given the extenuating circumstances their hands were tied.

Universal Credit

The numbers claiming this benefit escalated as not everyone qualified for furlough or self-employed compensation. Those on universal credit benefit were allocated a £20 per week "top up".

Unknown

So much about this virus was, and in some elements still is, unknown e.g., its origins, treatment, composition etc. As scientists obtain more insight and knowledge about the virus, they become aware of new mutations and variants, leading to more effective treatments.

Unprecedented

This is the ultimate and appropriate word to describe the havoc wreaked by this virus. The effects of plagues and wars pale into insignificance when witnessing its unrelenting path of global suffering and hardship. Coronavirus has changed lives forever and could be with us for years to come.

V

Vacancies

Job vacancies were at an all-time low. Those who had lost their jobs struggled to find re-employment.

Vaccine

The race was on all over the world to find a vaccine which is the only effective weapon to combat the virus. In November 2020 there was significant vaccine news. The front runners in the race were:

- PFIZER-BIONTECH – This vaccine was developed by a husband-and-wife team Ugur Sahin and his wife Oezlem. It injects genetic code into a fat droplet to instruct the body to make the Coronavirus spike protein so that the body can recognise and fight it. After final trial results and safety data it was rolled out in December 2020. The vaccine is difficult to transport and store as extremely low temperatures are required.

- ASTRA ZENECA – A vaccine developed by an Oxford team with Astra Zeneca. It uses a deactivated chimpanzee cold virus which triggers cells to produce the Coronavirus "Spike" protein. Favourable final trial results and safety data meant that this vaccine could also be rolled out December 2020. It is easy to transport and store as extreme temperatures are not required.

- MODERNA – Manufactured in America. Works in the same way as the Pfizer vaccine. Reports indicating its safety meant that it would be in use April 2021.

Two other vaccines are undergoing safety trials:

- JANSSEN – Works like the Oxford vaccine.
- NOVAVAX – Contains a synthesised copy of the Covid spike protein and an immune booster.

The advent of these vaccines triggered a rise in shares, particularly aviation, on the stock markets (SEE EFFICACY-ANTI-VACCINE)

Vaccine Passports

There are on-going discussions about these being a requirement for travel and entry into pubs and restaurants. This suggestion is beset with logistical and ethical problems. Vaccine passports are not feasible until everyone has been vaccinated. An alternative is proof of a negative Covid test.

Variant

Coronavirus has mutated. This happens with all viruses. The variant spreads more rapidly but it is not thought to cause greater illness. It will be halted by vaccines. News of the Kent variant in the UK caused other countries to refuse entry to the British. The channel port of Dover was closed for two days. There were long tailbacks. Drivers had to be tested before crossings resumed. Other variants are the Brazilian, South African, and Indian.

Vector

The carrier of a disease or infection.

Ventilators

During the first wave of the Pandemic ventilators were used to aid breathing as the virus attacked the lungs. The supply became short and innovative designs were manufactured and introduced. (SEE FORMULA ONE)

Veterans

A great number of veterans came forward to give aid wherever it was required.

Vilanterol

A drug used in the treatment of Coronavirus. It is a Bronchodilator prescribed and used to widen the bronchioles and improve breathing.

Virology

Members of the Institute of Virology appeared on TV etc. to expound their thoughts and theories about the virus.

Virus

A very simple micro-organism which can replicate itself within living cells causing disease.

Visors

Use of visors by doctors, dentists, chiropodists, and hairdressers etc. gave an added safety measure along with the use of masks. The use of visors is helpful when communicating with the deaf.

Vogue Cover

For the June 2020 issue of Vogue magazine photographs of frontline workers were displayed. This was another means of expressing gratitude to them.

Volunteers

People from all walks of life came forward to offer their help in a variety of ways. A wonderful sense of community spirit was in evidence. (SEE VETERANS)

Vulnerable

People with underlying illnesses were particularly susceptible to the virus. During the first lockdown, the government sent letters to them urging them to "shield" and not to venture out.

W

Walking

During lockdown exercising out of doors was permitted. Many people took this opportunity to go for daily walks locally in parks and beauty spots. New environmental locations were discovered and appreciated.

Waving

Relatives and friends were not allowed to visit homes, care homes, or hospitals. They could only wave to relatives and friends at windows from outside.

Webinars (aka Seminars)

Seminars have been conducted over the Internet via ZOOM.

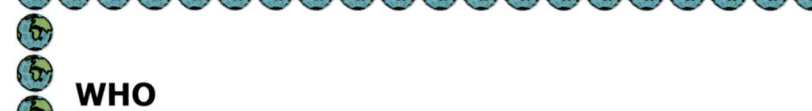

WHO

The World Health Organisation has played its part in this global Pandemic.

Wildlife

Wildlife has benefited and flourished during lockdown as there have been less people, vehicles, machinery, and pollution about. Some species have become more daring and ventured out of their normal habitats to explore others.

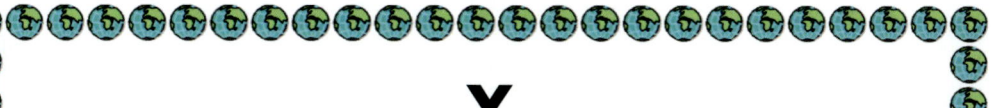

X

X-Rays

X-Rays have been invaluable in determining the effects of Covid-19 on the body, particularly the lungs.

Y

Yellow Card System

The MRHA devised this system in its quest to have pharmacological vigilance. Professionals and lay people are encouraged to submit findings good or bad concerning drugs and living organisms.

Youth

The young have been most vulnerable socially and economically during the Pandemic. The following are areas of most concern because of adverse effects:

1. Education

During the first lockdown, schools, colleges, and universities were closed. The importance of education and the fact that the virus does not affect the young too badly meant that schools, colleges, and universities re-opened as it was a priority to keep them open. Unfortunately, two further lockdowns ensued. Places of learning closed and did not re-open until March 2021

2. Housing

Many young people have lost their jobs and have been unable to pay their rent. (SEE LANDLORDS AND MORTGAGE HOLIDAYS)

3. Unemployment and redundancy

Unemployment and redundancy were rife among the young.

Z

Zoom

Video conferencing calls have been an invaluable means of communication during the Pandemic.

Zoonotic Viruses

Diseases that can jump from animals to humans.

Zoos

Zoos were closed. No visitors therefore no income. The animals still had to be fed and cared for – vets bills, heating, maintenance of buildings, payment of zookeepers etc. It was a difficult time and survival was an issue. On the brighter side there have been births e.g., baby Rhino.

107